THE PENIS BOOK

The penis book

An owner's manual

Margaret Gore

ALLEN & UNWIN

First published in 1997 by
Allen & Unwin
9 Atchison Street
St Leonards NSW 2065
Australia
Phone: (61 2) 8425 0100
Fax: (61 2) 9906 2218
E-mail: frontdesk@allen-unwin.com.au
URL: http://www.allen-unwin.com.au

National Library of Australia
Cataloguing-in-Publication entry:

Gore, Margaret, 1948– .
    The penis book: an owner's manual.

    ISBN 1 86448 329 6.

    1. Penis—Care and hygiene. 2. Generative organs, Male—
    Care and hygiene. 3. Men—Health and hygiene. 4. Men—
    Physiology. 5. Sex instruction for men. I. Title.

613.952

Set in 11/14pt NewBaskerville by DOCUPRO, Sydney
Printed and bound by Australian Print Group, Maryborough, Vic.

10 9 8 7 6 5 4 3 2

Contents

Acknowledgements   *viii*

Introduction   *ix*

1 Sex, lies and video tapes   **1**
   Myths   *1*
   Sexual performance   *11*

**2 The plumbing—How the penis and
   testes work**   **14**
   The mechanics   *14*
   Fertility   *17*
   Circumcision   *18*
   Maintenance   *18*

3 Puberty blues   **20**
   Your changing shape   *20*
   Wet dreams   *22*
   Masturbation   *23*
   Orgasm   *24*
   Sexuality   *25*

4 Contraception for men   **27**
   The condom   *27*

Periodic abstinence 29
Withdrawal 30
Vasectomy 31
Non-penetrative sex 31
Methods that don't work 32

5 What you should know about HIV/AIDS 33

6 Other sexually transmitted diseases 38
Syphilis 39
Gonorrhoea 40
Non-specific urethritis 41
Chlamydia 42
Genital herpes 43
Genital warts 45
Hepatitis B 46
Thrush 48
Trichomoniasis 48
Pubic lice 49
Scabies 50

**7 What happens when you go to a sexual
health centre 51**
The interview 52
The examination 54
Treatment 56
What is safe sex? 57
What is unsafe sex? 58

8 Sexual problems and solutions 59
Lack of sexual desire 59
Premature ejaculation 63
Impotence 65
Penile implants 69
Drug injections 70

9 Sex as you grow older 71
Community attitudes 72
Physical changes in men 73

Medical problems   75

**10 The most commonly asked questions
     about sex**   78

Glossary   84

Acknowledgements

The author gratefully acknowledges the assistance of the following authorities in the writing of this book: Dr John Horvath, Royal Prince Alfred Hospital; Dr Edith Weisberg, Medical Director, Family Planning Association of NSW; Professor Roger Short, Department of Physiology, Monash University; Dr E. T. Butterworth; Ms Margaret Winn, Health Educator, AIDS Education Unit, NSW Department of Health; Ms Jo Sexton, HIV Services Coordinator, NSW Health Services Development Unit; Sydney Sexual Health Centre, Sydney Hospital; Health Promotions Division, NSW Department of Health; Dr Sue Carruthers.

Note

This book is not a substitute for medical diagnosis or treatment. We advise you to always consult your doctor if you have any concerns about your health or for specific information regarding a personal medical matter.

Introduction

From the day you're born to the day you die you are a sexual being—it's inescapable—and although society prefers to think of children and old people as asexual, the truth is that sexuality is an essential part of your nature. A man's genitalia are not simply reproductive organs but the symbol of his manhood; they can be the source of great pleasure but, sadly, also of confusion and anxiety.

You may have many concerns—about penis size, sexual frequency, number of partners and your performance as a lover. You may be curious about whether you 'do it' like other men; if they go off sex from time to time as you do; if your fantasies are normal; if you masturbate too much; whether not liking oral or anal sex makes you weird.

Although men talk a lot about sex, they're not open and honest about the reality of their experiences, so they can't learn from one another. Most are too embarrassed to buy or borrow books on the subject, and so remain in agonising ignorance.

Because sex is such a fundamentally intimate subject and tied so closely to manhood and self-esteem, men are reluctant to seek help and so small worries build to deeper anxieties, which simply compound the problem.

Answer these questions: Would you ask your friends, partner or doctor for sex advice? If you did, would you feel it was an admission of inadequacy that left you open to ridicule? If you answered 'no' to the first and 'yes' to the second question, you're not alone, most men would answer the same way. As a result, you live with a sense of isolation caused by this sexual ignorance, little realising that you're all trying to conquer the same fears, and while you are all quite different, with different needs and desires, your quest for the truth about sex is the same.

Since this book was first published in 1991, there has been a rash of texts and television programs devoted to the subject of sex. But rather than being enlightening, these have contributed to the confusion, creating mixed messages when combined with the mass of explicit novels, movies and videos which have also burgeoned during this time. It's hardly surprising that many men have difficulty recognising fact from fiction.

Contributing to men's anxiety is the fact that women have a high sexual expectation these days. The mechanics of sex are discussed almost weekly in women's magazines—'how to have multiple orgasms', 'how to get horny', 'are you getting enough from your man?', 'what to do if he has a headache'. In the 1990s, women are expected to feel randy, be easily aroused and have multiple orgasms. All this puts pressure on a man to perform well, be a good lover and give her orgasms. Before the sexual revolution of the 1960s, women had little knowledge of sex and 'put up' with it for their marriages' sake. Men were considered good lovers if they were gentle, understanding, and 'quick', in consideration of their wife. If she didn't like his lovemaking, it was her problem, not his. Once women became liberated and knowledgeable, however, men had to lift their game and are now expected to use a range of sexual techniques and positions and enjoy experimentation with toys. It's no wonder many men are tuning out, turning off and going to sleep at night!

This book is designed to help you understand more about the reality of sex, and to provide practical information about your body—how it works and what to do if things go wrong, how to have a better sexual relationship with your partner and how the nature of your sexuality will change through the years. We hope it will allay your fears, correct misconceptions and lead to a more physically and emotionally satisfying life.

1
Sex, lies and video tapes

How do men learn about sex? From whom do they get their information? Although there has been an improvement in sex education in recent years, there are still many men who learn about sex through schoolyard jokes, erotic fiction and pornographic magazines and videos. These portray a totally unrealistic view of sex and perpetuate the myths about penis size, sexual performance and what it takes to be a 'man'.

First, let's look at the seven myths of male sexuality that prevent men from developing their sexual potential and from enjoying nurturing and satisfying relationships.

MYTHS

Myth number 1: 'I've got a dick that's two feet long, hard as steel and can go all night'

No matter what size of penis a man has, he still has nagging doubts that it isn't big enough. From the time he was a small boy, he has been surreptitiously comparing his penis with those of other males. In the locker room, or at the urinal, he has been asking the question, 'Is mine as big as his?'.

Fuelling this concern is the 'mythical penis' which only comes in three sizes—huge, gigantic and so large you can't get it through the door! Fiction and films are great reinforcers of this myth and it's surprising that popular, intelligent authors such as Harold Robbins and Henry Miller, not to mention the likes of Jackie Collins, are guilty of sustaining it.

In works of fiction the penis is forever 'a blood-gorged pole of muscle', 'throbbing', 'pulsating', 'hard as steel', 'springing swollen into her hands'. The same is true of porno films and magazines. The men are always of 'huge' proportions, with rigid erections that last for hours. The penis is always there, 'ready, willing and able' to leap forth into action as soon as a man's fly is unzipped.

Let's look at the facts: there are no muscles in the penis, it cannot vibrate, and quite often it's content to stay happily out of sight. If you could only see what happens on the film or photographic set and the reels of film that end up on the cutting room floor! Getting 'the star' hard is often difficult in the first place, and collapsing erections regularly ruin a scene, but you never see this on film. Clever camera angles and astute cutting ensures that the stud's willie is 'a rampant tool of infinite power'. Sure, there are a few men with out-sized penises (in most cases it's their only claim to fame) and they are eagerly sought out by the porn industry, but they are statistically rare. Flaccid penises do vary in size, but the difference evens out substantially when the penis becomes erect. Studies in America and Japan have revealed that the average-sized erect penis is about 13.5 centimetres. One study in Japan showed that out of 2300 men who were measured, only six were under 9 centimetres and only six recorded 20 centimetres.

However, from cradle to grave, men are convinced that a big dick is important to their masculinity. With all this propaganda, it's no wonder they feel their 'real life' penis is not long enough, wide enough or hard enough, that it does not spring forth with the appropriate attitude, and that it lacks stamina. The myth is so ingrained in the male psyche that it is very hard to shift.

You've probably read the above and said, 'Yeah, yeah, but I *really* know that a big dick makes you a man'. As long as you compare your penis size and sexual performance with the mythical penis, you are going to feel sexually anxious.

So why is size unimportant? Well, let's look at the female anatomy. First, it is the outer third of the vagina that contains nerve endings that are sensitive to touch. The inner two-thirds are relatively insensitive. (If a woman had more nerve endings in this area she would never have more than one child because childbirth would be so painful.) Stimulation to the outer third of the vagina is what counts. A large penis is really surplus to requirements.

Second, most women attain a greater sexual arousal by having their clitoris stimulated, rather than just vaginal thrusting by a penis. You would have to have an L-shaped penis to be inside the vagina and stimulate the clitoris with it at the same time. Some women do experience orgasm through penile penetration but, remember, it is in the outer third of the vagina where they feel the sensation. The thrusting of the penis also pulls on the vaginal lips which are attached to the clitoral hood and this too can produce orgasm. Many women who don't have orgasms during intercourse, can do so when they or their partners stimulate the clitoris. So, here again, penis size is not a factor.

It's also important to understand that the vagina is not a 'hole' in the woman's body. In an unaroused state the walls of the vagina lie together. It's an area of great elasticity, that can accommodate any size from a finger to a baby. When sexually aroused the vagina becomes more elastic in order to receive the penis and will form itself snugly around whatever size of penis is inserted. So again, size is really just not that big a deal. It's more 'how' you make love, rather than your penis size that counts.

Men sometimes also worry that the size of their penis will affect their fertility. Forget it—it has no bearing on your ability to father children.

Myth number 2: 'Me Tarzan . . . you Jane'
This is a complicated one because it combines the contradictory notions that men should be in charge

of sex with the idea that women are now the sexual predators.

On the one hand many men feel that they should initiate sex and be in charge of the 'performance'. They cling to the notion that being a man means being dominant, and not being in charge is a sign of weakness. The trouble with this attitude is that it totally excludes the woman's desires. Consequently, men miss out on the real joy of sex, the comfort and reassurance of intimacy and the confidence that comes from being truly in touch with themselves.

On the other hand, women are now more assertive about their sexual needs, and their desire to be an active partner in sex. They have acquired the confidence to express what they want. Some men find this threatening because, in many ways, it's calling their bluff—they might not be able to meet their partner's demands, or live up to their expectations. When women didn't have any sexual expectations, it was easy for the man to satisfy himself without concern for the woman.

It's important to realise that it's all right to take both the active and the passive role during sex; it doesn't make you less of a man or diminish you in the eyes of your partner. Many men tell sex counsellors they would like more help from their partner, that they don't like 'playing in the dark'. Unfortunately, few are able to communicate this. What you should realise is that women feel like this too and would like to talk more about sex. Try discussing it with your partner and see how she responds—you'll be pleasantly surprised.

Learning to be more passive and letting your partner stimulate you the way you like is also important if you have trouble getting or maintaining an erection. It allows you to concentrate on your own sensations, which can often overcome the lack of, or a not fully firm, erection as well as increasing the pleasure for both of you.

A good lover is confident, relaxed and uninhibited. He takes his time over sex, is sensitive to his partner's needs, is prepared to talk to her about what turns her on and is able to tell her what he enjoys. It is a close, intimate, mutually satisfying experience.

Myth number 3: 'Sex means intercourse'

Good sex doesn't have to end up with a penis in a vagina. In fact, with good sex, penile penetration of the vagina is only one aspect of the total experience. It may surprise you, but just as a woman does not need a penis in her vagina, nor an orgasm to get sexual satisfaction, *neither do you.* It's a very blinkered view that says orgasms, and the more the better, are the be all and end all of sex. Once you get rid of this notion, you'll be able to enjoy a broader range of personal and sexual relationships.

It's very important to consider your attitude to sex and particularly to 'foreplay'. Is it just something you have to go through to get to the main event—intercourse? Is it a question of a standard procedure to be followed before you're allowed in? Or are you really enjoying touching your partner's body, savouring the intimacy of the experience? Perhaps we should change the word 'foreplay' to 'sex play' because this might help dispel the idea that touching, caressing, oral sex and masturbation are just steps to go through before the 'biggy'—penetration.

Orgasm can bring pleasure, but without an appreciation of intimacy, sensitivity and, above all, sensuality, sex is little more than a biological function. In Western cultures, sensitivity and sensuality have been so successfully divorced from our sexuality, that for a great many people true intimacy in sexual relationships is never achieved.

There is immense satisfaction to be gained from closeness, cuddling, kissing, stroking and fondling, as well as oral sex and mutual masturbation. There are so many other things to enjoy in sex than just 'ramming it in and banging away'. Learning to be intimate with your partner may not come easily to you, but if you try, you will find that it not only brings great joy but eases loneliness and makes you feel good about yourself.

Myth number 4: 'Physical contact must always lead to intercourse'

This is a sad one because it deprives both you and your partner of a close physical bond that has little to do with sex. In porno movies and erotic fiction, people never cuddle, kiss, hug, stroke or fondle their partner without it leading quickly to intercourse. Yet this denies that human beings need physical closeness with the people they care about. Our cultural upbringing has taught men to show their emotions rarely and so places them in an emotional straitjacket. You may have broken free, but others remain totally at a loss as to how to deal with their feelings.

Touching, stroking, caressing are all comforting and reassuring gestures from one human being to another. We all understand how much babies and young children need this close physical contact and we suppose, wrongly, that we grow out of it. It's true that most of us don't need the same degree of physical reassurance as a young child, but we do need physical affection in our lives.

If you can say to your partner, 'Look, darling, I don't feel like sex tonight, but I would love a cuddle', you'll have a closer and more rewarding relationship.

Being held in someone's arms, without any other demands being made, is a great antidote to stress; being stroked is soothing, having your breasts or penis fondled (without sexual intent) is a loving, caring and intimate experience.

Unfortunately, many men consider this kind of touching as 'teasing' and won't touch their partner or allow themselves to be touched unless the intention is intercourse. Small wonder, then, that their relationships are two dimensional and they have needs they can't express.

Try talking to your partner about the way you

actually feel, and listen to what she tells you about her feelings. You'll probably find that instead of clinging to opposite sides of the bed, you can find a comfort zone in the middle.

Myth number 5: 'Men are always ready for sex'

The truth is that men do not always want sex, and while we are one of only a few animals with the potential to have sex at any time, we are still tied to biological rhythms that govern our moods and desires. If you believe you should be 'ready, willing and able' to have sex whenever the opportunity arises, you'll worry if you can't rise to the occasion, and if this happens two or three times, you may worry that you'll never feel like it again—it's the old idea of 'Use it or lose it'. However, you are subject to mental and emotional influences just as a woman is. You are also placed under a great deal of stress in today's world. There is pressure to perform well and achieve in work, in sport, and in sex. And just as some days you'd rather not be at work, and sometimes your sporting performance is not up to scratch, there will be times when you just don't feel like sex. There is nothing wrong with you, it's not an early sign of impotence, and you're not having a mental breakdown. It's perfectly normal. Every man will experience this at some time or another, it's just that nobody admits it. Traditionally, it was the woman who made the excuses but today men are having 'headaches', or 'having to get up early in the morning'. Just be honest with your partner.

Say something like, 'I don't feel like sex, but that doesn't mean I don't love you or want to be close to you'.

Myth number 6: 'Sex requires an erection'

Let's say it again, loud and clear, there's more to sex than putting a penis into a vagina. Seeing sex only in terms of intercourse narrows the experience for both partners and the relationship may never become fulfilling for either.

This myth brings us back to our fantasy world where the penis is the star of the show. Does it mean that if the star fails to turn up, the show is cancelled? Sadly, if you believe that sex requires an erection this is the case, which leaves both you and your partner frustrated and disappointed.

Many couples have discovered that there is a lot of sex play that doesn't require an erection and enjoy mutually satisfying sex lives. Stimulation to a flaccid penis can still feel great. A massage can be sensual and sexual, as can oral sex—the experience is limited only by your imagination. Of course, talking it over with your partner will help. You could say something like, 'I don't think Willie is going to show up tonight, but we can still have fun without him'. You never know, you may be having such a good time that he doesn't want to miss out.

Penises can be oddly perverse at times and seem to have a mind of their own. If its importance is ignored, and you just get on and have some fun, it often joins the party. Conversely, if you are so worried about getting it up, and focus on your lack of erection, then it will perversely stay comatose.

It is also important for disabled men to realise that they can still enjoy sex, even if they can't have an erection and/or experience intercourse. The elderly don't need to give up the joys of sex either because of impotence problems (see Chapter 8).

Myth number 7: 'We're so enlightened these days that nobody believes these myths any more'

The main reason for producing this book was the number of letters that pour in from men to medical columns in magazines requesting sex information. Letters from bewildered teenagers, confused twenty-year-olds, frightened middle-aged men, the anxious elderly, all testify to the fact that the myths are as ingrained as ever.

SEXUAL PERFORMANCE

First and foremost, sex is not a performance, nor a competition, nor a race. Sex is a mutually satisfying, physical intimacy between people. However, men today are under pressure to excel in everything they do including sex. They take their responsibilities very seriously, to the extent that they regard themselves as being responsible not only for their own orgasms but for their partner's too.

The first lesson to learn is that nobody can make another person have an orgasm. Whether a woman gets to that point of arousal where she has an orgasm depends on what is going on in her head at the time. Of course, it's important that you give her the right sort of stimulation, but if you are and she still doesn't 'come', it's not your fault. Perhaps she has other things on her mind which makes her unreceptive to orgasm. It doesn't mean that she is not enjoying your lovemaking—she just doesn't have an orgasm.

Sex shouldn't have a goal, such as intercourse and orgasm—it's simply for giving and getting pleasure. You don't have to pursue the 'Holy Grail' of orgasm from point A to point B in the shortest possible time. Taking your time, being relaxed and simply enjoying what you and your partner are doing to one another, will give you both a great deal more pleasure than turning the experience into an Olympic event. You could stop halfway through, enjoy a glass of wine and a snack, have a bath or shower, go for a swim, still enjoying touching, cuddling and kissing, then continue afterwards.

Once you get away from the idea that 'penis in vagina' is the ultimate in sex, you relieve an enormous amount of pressure. A woman can lie there and be totally non-aroused, have intercourse and pretend that she's having a good time. You can't do that, because the lack of an erection is pretty obvious. And if that's the be all and end all of being a man, it's a humiliating experience.

By removing that pressure you'll have a much better chance of getting closer to each other, because you're not trying to reach the 'magical goal' of orgasm. You'll stop trying for a 'massive' erection that is going to give her a 'wonderful' orgasm. Of course, you should enjoy intercourse, but don't see it as the ultimate sexual activity.

2
The plumbing— How the penis and testes work

THE MECHANICS

Although you handle your penis and balls every day, you may not know exactly how they work. A man's genitalia consists of the penis and the scrotum, which is the loose bag that hangs down behind the penis. You may think that men only have external sex organs, but like women men also have internal sex organs. They consist of the testes (also called testicles), vasa deferentia, seminal vesicles, Cowper's glands, prostate gland and urethra (see diagram on next page).

The testes lie inside the scrotum, commonly called 'balls'. In fact, your balls are not solid lumps as you might expect but are made up of a mass of tiny tubes which, if stretched out, would be longer than two or three football fields! One testis, usually the left, hangs lower than the other and some men worry about whether this is normal or not—it is.

Figure 2.1 Male reproductive organs

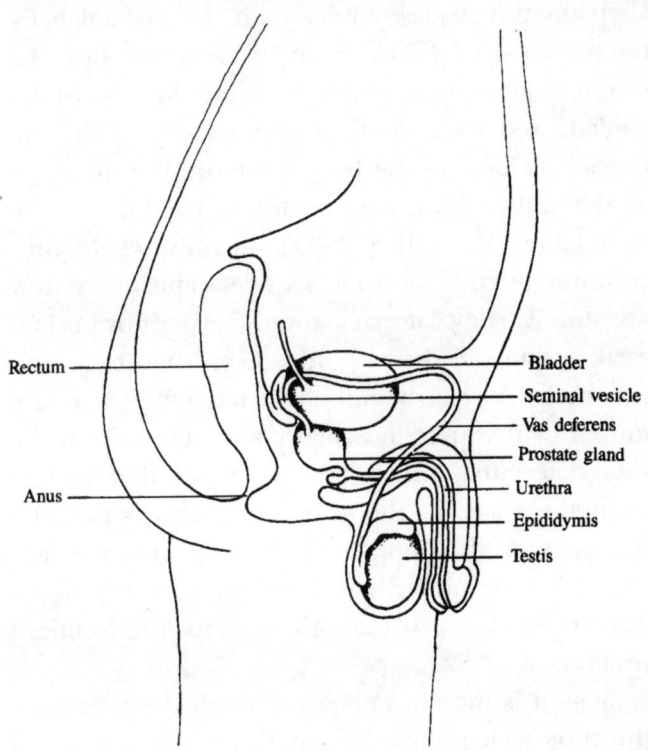

Rectum

Anus

Bladder
Seminal vesicle
Vas deferens
Prostate gland
Urethra
Epididymis
Testis

It's in the testes that sperm are made in huge quantities—one ejaculation will contain as many as 400 million. You may think that semen and sperm are the same thing, but they're not. Sperm makes up only about 1 per cent of the fluid that you ejaculate.

Your testes manufacture sperm constantly at the rate of around 100 million per day. To keep this sperm factory manufacturing efficiently, your body has to regulate the temperature of the testes, and keep them a degree cooler than the normal body temperature of 37°C. If the weather is hot the scrotum allows the testes to hang loosely to be cooled, and on cold days, the scrotum pulls the testes up closer to the body for more warmth.

When the sperm have been produced they move to a large tube called the epididymis, where they continue to grow for up to six weeks and where they are stored ready for ejaculation. During this period, weak sperm will die off and be absorbed back into the body. At ejaculation the surviving sperm are moved by rhythmic muscular contractions down the vasa deferentia, which are two tubes that extend from the testes to the seminal vesicles. When the sperm reach the upper end of these tubes they are mixed with seminal fluid, which is a secretion produced by the prostate gland and the seminal vesicles.

Semen is then ejaculated through the urethra—the tube which runs the length of your penis and which you urinate through. However, when your penis is erect, a tiny valve closes the urethra off from the bladder to prevent semen from mixing with any urine. This is the reason you can't pee when you have a hard-on.

It's a good idea to get into the habit of examining your testes regularly. The best time is after a warm shower or bath, when your scrotum is more relaxed. Gently roll each testis between your thumb and fingers. It should feel smooth, egg-shaped and free of any lumps, without any unusually sensitive areas. The reason for doing this is because cancer of the testes accounts for between 1–2 per cent of all male cancers and is almost always curable if caught early enough. Since this form of cancer affects men mostly in their 20s and 30s, you should make this a regular monthly routine—just as a woman should examine her breasts. If you notice any changes, or lumps or soreness, then see your doctor.

The penis consists of the shaft, head (known as the glans) and the foreskin in uncircumcised men. It contains no muscles, so you can't make it bigger with exercise. What it does consist of is a great many nerve endings and three cylindrical areas of spongy tissue contained in a tough fibrous covering. The penis is aroused when signals from the brain and spinal cord send blood flooding into these spongy cylinders. As they fill with blood, they press against the outer covering making your penis longer, wider and stiff. Your penis also extends far back into your body, almost to your rectum and you can feel this most noticeably when you have an erection. This area, too, can be sensitive to sexual stimulation. However, for many men it is the glans, or head, of the penis which is most sensitive, especially the ridge that joins the glans to the shaft, called the corona.

FERTILITY

Fertilisation takes place when a sperm reaches and penetrates a receptive egg. The sperm (100 million of them would be contained in a millilitre of semen) swim by propelling themselves forward by their tails, up through the vagina to the opening of the uterus, known as the cervix, then on through the womb to the fallopian tubes. If the woman has recently ovulated (produced an egg), the sperm will try to burrow into it and if one succeeds the egg is fertilised. No further sperm can then penetrate the egg. Sperm can live in a woman's body for a few days, so conception can occur some time after intercourse. It has been known for women to become pregnant without having intercourse, when sperm have been ejaculated at the opening of her vagina.

CIRCUMCISION

At birth, the head of the penis is covered with a hood of skin called the foreskin. Circumcision is an operation usually carried out on babies, where the foreskin is surgically removed. Being circumcised is not as common as it once was and is done for social or religious reasons rather than for health ones. Whether you are circumcised or not makes no difference to your sexuality or fertility.

MAINTENANCE

Keeping your genitals clean is important, especially if you are not circumcised. When you wash, pull back your foreskin and clean your glans thoroughly, because a cheesy-like substance called smegma is secreted by the tiny glands near the head of the penis; if the glans is not washed regularly you could develop an unpleasant odour and a painful infection of your penis as a consequence. Many women also get vaginal infections because of the poor hygiene of their sexual partners.

Keeping your genitalia in good working order is, of course, important for your physical and sexual well-being. Cleanliness, as I have just mentioned, is important but there are other aspects you should keep in mind.

Wearing tight underpants and jeans can prevent the scrotum from keeping the testes at the proper temperature for making sperm, which can affect your fertility. Also, tight clothing doesn't allow proper ventilation for your genital area and the subsequent hot and sweaty conditions can leave you prone to rashes and thrush. So be sensible about what you wear.

3
Puberty blues

Exactly when puberty occurs in boys is difficult to say except that it can begin as early as ten years old and end as late as eighteen years. The changes start earlier in some boys than others and can happen over a longer or shorter period. Everyone has their own individual internal clock for the timing of puberty. You might be one of the few who reach puberty by eleven, or someone who is just emerging from it about the time you're leaving school. You can't change this biological timing—you just have to accept it.

YOUR CHANGING SHAPE

When puberty begins, your body will undergo a number of changes, triggered by the release of sex hormones. The main male hormone is called testosterone and its effect is to prepare you for fathering children.

The first thing you'll notice is a sudden increase in the rate of growth of your testes and scrotum, followed by the appearance of coarse pubic hair which will start to grow around your genitals, in your armpits, on your chest and, eventually, on your face. (The amount of hair you grow is like everything else about you—hereditary—and some boys will have more than others.) Your penis will then become larger and more sensitive to touch, reaching its full adult size about two years later. You may also experience a slight enlargement of your breasts, but don't worry, it doesn't mean you're turning into a girl. It's a condition called gynaecomastia and is caused by the hormonal upheaval that's going on in your body at this time. It's quite normal, will soon pass and is experienced by about 80 per cent of pubescent boys.

Boys tend to become obsessed with sex during puberty and worry that they are turning into sex-crazed fiends. The truth is that your hormones are having such a strong influence on your body that it is almost impossible for you *not* to be obsessed with sex. When are you going to lose your virginity? Who are you going to have sex with? Will you know what to do? Will you be any good at it? What if you come before you 'get it in'? These questions go through every boy's mind during adolescence. Added to this sexual tension is the 'sure' knowledge that all your mates have already done it and that you're the last virgin on the block. Be assured, there are far more male teenage virgins out there than will ever be admitted.

Erections can be a real problem for pubescent boys as they seem to happen at the drop of a hat. You don't even have to be thinking about sex for one to pop up, which can be extremely embarrassing. You seem to have no control over your penis—it almost appears to have a mind of its own. This is quite normal and can be due to a number of things—tensions in your body, changes in temperature or motion like riding on a bus or train. It's best to ignore it, which we admit is easier said than done, but focusing on your erection will only make it harder and last longer. By taking your mind off it, it will probably disappear.

Although you may have experienced erections and orgasms before, the first time you ejaculate may come as quite a surprise, but it's a landmark in your growing up because it signals that you are now an adolescent. The first time you see or feel your own semen may also startle you. Semen is the thick, whitish fluid that spurts from your penis when you reach orgasm; its consistency can vary from boy to boy and in some it can appear almost lumpy. This is quite normal, but many boys think there is something wrong and that they may have a disease. Relax, it's only your body getting used to producing sperm and semen, everything will settle down in time.

WET DREAMS

These are a common occurrence in boys in their early teens. A wet dream is when you ejaculate in your sleep, although it can also happen during waking hours while day-dreaming. It is quite involuntary, but can cause shock and embarrassment. You may think you've wet the bed, or feel ashamed that you might have been having sexual fantasies. It's important to realise that it is a perfectly normal occurrence and you should not feel embarrassed if this happens to you.

MASTURBATION

Our ideas about masturbation have progressed greatly in the past few decades. It's no longer considered an unnatural act that will damage your health. It's sad to think of the misery boys with bad eyesight went through, because they believed the myth that masturbation made you blind! It's now recognised as a natural expression of the sexual development in children and adolescents, and as normal sexual activity during adulthood. It can relieve sexual tension, and also gives you the chance to discover the sensations of sex in a relaxed, private way. You'll discover what turns you on, how you like to be touched and what an ejaculation and orgasm feel like. You will also learn to recognise the 'point of no return', when ejaculation is inevitable, so that you can control when you want orgasm to occur. So long as it is done in private, you should not feel guilty about masturbating, but enjoy the feeling of exploring your own sexuality.

ORGASM

It's almost impossible to describe an orgasm. It's like describing a colour only you have seen, because orgasm is a different experience for everyone. We can describe mechanically what happens but it's impossible to tell you what it feels like.

Physically, an orgasm is the climax of a complex series of responses of the genital organs, caused by sexual excitement, commonly known as 'coming'. During sex play and intercourse there is a growing sense of sexual tension, which builds to an exciting point of release. Your breathing and heart rate will increase and your erection will seem to get even harder. The sexual tension will mount and then at the height of excitement, some of the muscles around the base of your penis will go into rhythmic contractions; there will be a feeling of tightening and relaxing of these muscle and it's at this point that you will ejaculate. After ejaculation, the muscles of your body will relax and you will go into what is called the refractory period, which is when your body recovers from the orgasm. The blood will flow from your penis back to the rest of your body and your penis will probably become limp, although this does not always happen immediately. During this refractory period you will not be able to have another erection. In teenagers this time of recuperation can be only a few minutes, but it tends to take longer to get back into sexual mode as you get older.

Generally women take longer to reach orgasm than men, so it is important to be caring, honest and sensitive to your partner's needs. If a woman is tense it will probably take her longer to reach orgasm, while you are likely to 'come' much faster. Read the chapters on male myths and sexual problems in this book to get a fuller understanding of what sex is all about. It might help to dispel some of your worries.

SEXUALITY

Sexuality is present in everyone from birth to death, but develops with increasing urgency during puberty. It's important that you understand your own sexuality and learn to feel comfortable with it. Many teenagers are unsure about sex and they can find the whole subject quite confusing, which isn't surprising when you realise that they are being influenced by their mates, parents, teachers and perhaps their Church, who all have opinions about sex and which are usually inconsistent.

Your mates' advice is 'as early and as often'. Your parents may hope you'll wait until you're older and meet the right girl. Each state and territory has different laws of consent. The Church may want you to be a virgin on your wedding night! Different cultures and age groups have differing ideas about when people should be allowed to have sex and who makes a suitable partner. This is why it's important for you to find out correct information about sex, so that you can make up your own mind. Your school or local library may have books about sex that you can read, or you could ask a counsellor at the Family Planning Association. This organisation helps not only those people who are planning a family, but also those who want to avoid pregnancy and sexually transmitted diseases (STDs), including single people and teenagers. You can ring for an appointment, then talk to one of their counsellors, alone or with your partner, about sexual facts, so that you can make good decisions about your sex life.

4
Contraception for men

If you're sexually active, or plan to be, and don't know much about contraception, now is the time to learn. It's important to discuss with your partner which method is going to suit you both best because it's a joint responsibility, no matter which of you actually uses the contraceptive. So don't just rely on your partner to take precautions—there are options for men, too.

THE CONDOM

With the high incidence of STDs and the chance of infected women becoming sterile for life, plus the threat of HIV/AIDS, condoms are now the contraceptive of first choice for all young couples starting sexual activity.

A condom is a fine rubber sheath which is worn on your erect penis, to collect sperm during ejaculation and stop it entering the vagina and uterus. It is 90–95 per cent effective if used correctly. It will

Figure 4.1 How to use a condom

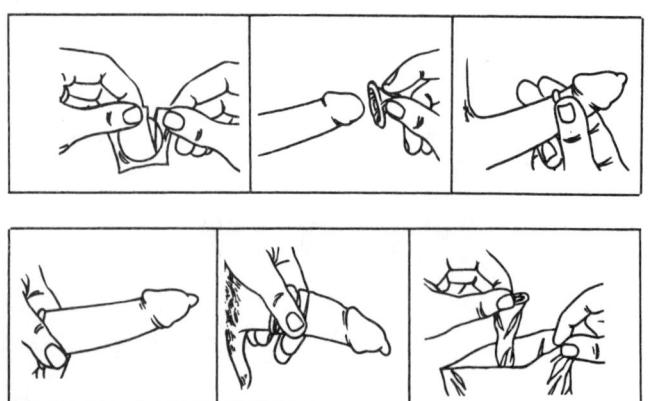

also give you protection from other sexually transmitted diseases, including HIV/AIDS, especially if
you use spermicidally lubricated condoms containing nonoxynol-9. However, a condom is only as good
as the person who uses it, and to make sure you
have maximum protection it is important that it is
put on and taken off correctly.

How to use a condom

- The condom must be placed on your erect penis
  before any sexual contact is made. To do this,
  roll the condom gently onto the penis all the way
  down to the base, leaving enough room at the
  tip to collect the semen. Some men make the
  mistake of pulling the condom on so tight that
  when they ejaculate the semen is squeezed down
  the sides and out from under the rim. Once the

condom is on your penis, squeeze the blind tip to expel any air trapped there.

- After ejaculation, hold the rim of the condom firmly at the base of your penis when withdrawing from the vagina, so that it does not slip off and spill semen onto the vagina—if this happens sperm can still swim up into the uterus.
- Wrap the condom in paper and dispose of it in the rubbish bin—not down the toilet.
- If you wish to use a lubricant with the condom, use only a water-based lubricant such as KY Jelly or Lubafax—not an oil-based one like Vaseline or baby oil. The oil will cause the rubber to deteriorate causing the condom to burst.
- Use a new condom every time you have intercourse.
- Don't keep condoms in a hot place as the rubber will perish. Buy condoms in foil packs as this protects against damage by UV light. Never use a condom that is more than two years old or older than its use-by date.

There are no side effects using this method of contraception. You can buy condoms from pharmacies, supermarkets, petrol stations, family planning clinics, vending machines and by mail order.

PERIODIC ABSTINENCE

Periodic abstinence means not having intercourse at a time of the month when your partner is likely to get pregnant. There are several ways a woman can tell when she is fertile such as the rhythm method, Billings (or mucus) method, calendar method and temperature method. If you and your partner choose one of these methods, you must be committed to making it work. This does not mean just abstaining from intercourse for a couple of days a month, but for a week or more. It's important that both you and your partner learn these techniques from a qualified family planning counsellor. Ask your doctor or local Family Planning Association for information.

WITHDRAWAL

'What do you call a man using the withdrawal method?'—'Daddy!' This joke may be old but it tells the truth—withdrawal is probably the least reliable method of contraception. Withdrawal (or coitus interruptus) is when you remove your penis from the vagina before ejaculation. This is the oldest form of contraception known in Biblical times as 'spilling the seed'. It is totally in your control and you must be very responsible as it is a risky method of con- traception. You may forget to withdraw when close to orgasm, or you may not be quick enough. It's important that you have enough control not to ejaculate while your penis is in your partner's vagina. There is also the risk that you may have already released thousands of sperm into her vagina—and it only takes one to make a baby—before ejacula- tion. If using this method it's also important not to ejaculate or spill semen on or near her genital area, because the sperm may still swim into the vagina— they're such determined little critters!

VASECTOMY

Vasectomy is the sterilisation of a man. As we saw in Chapter 2, sperm are produced in the testes and travel to the penis via the vasa deferentia. These tubes can be surgically cut and tied so that when a man ejaculates there are no sperm in his semen. Having a vasectomy is a simple operation which can be carried out in a clinic or surgery using only a local anaesthetic. An incision about 1–2 centimetres long is made in the upper side of the scrotum. The tubes lie just beneath the skin where they can be cut and sealed off.

Contraception is not effective immediately with this method because there may still be some sperm left in the tubes. It can take up to 16 ejaculations before the tubes are clear of sperm and a sperm count should be done at this time to check if the vasectomy has been successful. Although vasectomy is sometimes reversible, it should be viewed as irreversible when making the decision to have the operation.

NON-PENETRATIVE SEX

Remember, you don't have to have intercourse to enjoy sex. Touching, petting, kissing, stroking, mutual masturbation and oral sex are all ways of enjoying sex with your partner without intercourse. Like the withdrawal method, however, it is important that none of your semen gets near your partner's vagina because the race might be on that could lead to a pregnancy.

METHODS THAT DON'T WORK

There are many stories about how you can 'do it' without getting pregnant, like holding your breath when you partner 'comes', doing it standing up, sneezing before or after sex, jumping up and down after intercourse, and douching. Some young people also believe that women can't get pregnant the first time they have intercourse. Lies, lies and more lies. They can and probably will unless you get advice and use a safe contraceptive method. Ask your local GP or, if you want more anonymity, go to your local Family Planning Clinic, where the counsellors will be able to explain what options are available to you and what would best suit your needs.

5
What you should know about HIV/AIDS

Human Immunodeficiency Virus (HIV) attacks certain white blood cells in the human body, damaging the immune system and causing Acquired Immune Deficiency Syndrome (AIDS). As a consequence, the body becomes vulnerable to infections and diseases which it would normally fight off easily.

Although there has been a lot of media coverage about HIV/AIDS over the past decade, there are still many people who believe it's not a problem they have to worry about. The truth is that unless you are celibate (i.e. have no sexual contact with another person), or have been in a mutually faithful relationship since 1979, or know the HIV status of your partner, you may be at risk.

HIV is transmitted when semen, blood or vaginal fluids pass directly from an infected person to their sexual partner, by sharing needles and syringes, from an infected mother to her baby through breast milk, or by accident through needle stick injuries. Contrary to popular belief HIV/AIDS is not just a problem for the gay community, prostitutes or drug users. If you don't know the HIV status of the partners you're having sex with and are not practising safer sex techniques, you are putting yourself at risk. You can't catch the virus through ordinary social contact in public, at work or school. Nor can you catch it by shaking hands, ordinary social kissing, through food or normal everyday activities.

There is no set pattern to the development of this disease and as it can have a long incubation period, some HIV positive people may have no symptoms for many years, while others sadly develop full-blown AIDS and usually die within a few years of contracting the disease. The average time of infection to AIDS is 10 years.

Symptoms include:

- significant and unexplained weight loss of more than 4–5 kilos
- swollen lymph glands
- fever and night sweats
- persistent diarrhoea.

When a person has these symptoms they are said to have AIDS Related Complex (ARC) or Lymphadenopathy Syndrome (LAS). If the disease progresses to the terminal stage, the person's immune system is so badly damaged that they succumb to 'opportunistic infections' or other conditions which are rarely found in those with healthy immune systems.

Everyone should assess their own risk of contracting HIV/AIDS and adopt or maintain safer sexual and drug using practices. For example:

1 Develop a mutually monogamous relationship, which means having a faithful, one-to-one relationship, and where each partner is uninfected. Both partners must also avoid any risk-taking behaviour outside the relationship.

2 If you have several sexual partners, or if you are unsure of the HIV status of your partner, use safer sex practices. This means:

• Not allowing semen, vaginal fluid or blood to pass from one partner to the other. Using a condom provides a barrier against the transmission of the HIV virus during vaginal or anal intercourse. Anal intercourse is the most likely way to transmit the virus, particularly if the insertive partner is HIV positive and the recipient is HIV negative. It's important that condoms are worn correctly (see Chapter 4) to provide maximum protection.

• Being careful during mutual masturbation to ensure there are no cuts or sores on either partner's hands, penis or vagina and not using seminal or vaginal fluids as a lubricant. If using your fingers or hand in the vagina or anus, wear a latex glove for protection. Always change gloves when changing partners or moving from the anus to the vagina; and use plenty of water-based lubricant such as Wetstuff, KY Jelly or Glyde on the outside of the glove.

- Taking precautions during oral sex including fellatio (contact between the mouth and the penis), cunnilingus (contact between the mouth and the vagina), and rimming (contact between the mouth and the anus). Oral sex without ejaculation holds some risk of transferring HIV from the penis or vagina to the mouth of the other partner, but taking semen, vaginal fluids or blood into the mouth will increase that risk. If your mouth and throat are in perfect health then it's hard for HIV to be transmitted, but if you have gums that bleed, mouth ulcers, or any other infections or disease then you should take extra precautions. Remember that small cuts and bleeding gums can be caused by tooth brushing, flossing, throat infections or eating sharp foods such as corn chips, and you might not be aware you have injured your mouth. To check, rinse with warm salty water: if it stings, or you have known mouth disease, then use protection such as condoms for fellatio and dams (thin squares of latex) for cunnilingus and rimming. HIV is not easily transmitted by rimming, but many other serious illnesses like hepatitis A and B, intestinal germs and parasites are easily passed on this way. Using a dam helps guard against these infections.

- Using condoms on sex toys such as vibrators, dildos or buttplugs. Don't share toys during sex as it is possible for semen, vaginal fluids or blood to be passed from one partner to another. If moving toys from anus to vagina, use a new condom each time.

If you are at all concerned about your HIV status—a simple blood test will indicate if you are infected with HIV or not—consult your doctor, state AIDS Council or local sexual health centre (the number is in the front of the telephone book) who provide free, confidential testing and counselling (see Chapter 7).

6
Other sexually transmitted diseases

As the name implies, a sexually transmitted disease (STD) is any infection transmitted by sexual contact. Anyone who is sexually active, has more than one partner or is not in a monogamous relationship (i.e. where both partners have no other sexual contacts) is at risk of contracting an STD. Some of the infections we discuss in this chapter have no apparent symptoms, while others can range from a slight genital irritation to sores and rashes on different parts of the body. Some STDs can cause female infertility and cancer and, of course, today there is also HIV/AIDS to worry about (see Chapter 5).

Contrary to popular mythology, you can't tell if someone has an STD simply by looking at them. It's surprising how many young men still believe that the way a girl looks will show whether she is 'clean' or not. STDs don't respect class or economic background. Patients at STD clinics range from teen-agers to pensioners, barristers to shop assistants, prostitutes to politicians. So, if you're sexually active it's important to understand what the different STDs are, what, if any, are the symptoms, how they are treated and how to prevent them.

SYPHILIS

Syphilis is thought by many to be a disease of the past but STD clinics see it often enough to know that it's still present in our community; and it's a life-threatening disease if left untreated.

Syphilis germs enter the body through tiny breaks in the skin and the disease is almost always con-tracted through sexual contact. As the sores can be out of sight, such as under the scrotum, in the vagina or rectum, and disappear of their own accord, many people can pass it on unwittingly to their partners. Even if they do notice a small sore, they may ignore it as it usually disappears in a few weeks. However, the disease hasn't gone away—there's just no visible evidence of it.

During its progress the syphilis germs attack the body's organs causing major tissue damage resulting in heart disease, brain damage, paralysis and event-ually death. Fortunately, it's rarely seen in its latter stages these days because it's usually picked up and treated early. This is mainly due to the fact that all people attending an STD clinic or going to their doctor for any STD test, will also be tested for syphilis. If it's detected it's treated on the spot with a course of antibiotics.

Syphilis can be contracted through oral and anal sex, as well as through penis–vagina intercourse. It can also be spread by accidental exposure to the infectious ulcer or rash, and can be passed on to an unborn child.

Syphilis is diagnosed by a blood test, and can be cured with a course of antibiotics. However, whatever damage the disease has caused to the body can't be repaired, so early detection is extremely important.

Once treated, the patient should only become sexually active again once their doctor has said it's safe to do so. After treatment, check-ups will be essential one month after treatment and then periodically for up to two years.

GONORRHOEA

Gonorrhoea, also known as the 'clap', the 'drip', 'Jack', and a 'dose', is the third most common STD in the Western world, after non-specific urethritis and chlamydia. The gonorrhoea bacterium can't exist outside the human body and is transmitted by direct contact during oral, vaginal and anal sex.

The first symptoms are a yellowish, pus-like discharge and/or a burning sensation when urinating. The symptoms can appear in differing degrees and may be so slight they go unnoticed. If the disease has been contracted through oral sex, you may experience a sore throat; if through anal sex, there might be itching in the rectum, or a slight discharge sometimes with blood, and mucous may be found coating the faeces. If left untreated, gonorrhoea can cause inflammation in many parts of the body, and spread to the testes, causing pain and some risk of infertility.

If you experience any of these symptoms, see your doctor immediately or go to a sexual health centre for tests (see Chapter 7). A swab of the secretions from the penis, throat or rectum will be taken (depending on the type of intercourse). The results of the tests will be ready in 10–15 minutes and if the disease is confirmed, you will be treated on the spot. Treatment usually consists of a one-off dose of antibiotics or penicillin. If you have picked up gonorrhoea in South-East Asia you will be treated with a non-penicillin drug, as the Asian strain is resistant to penicillin. It's important to have a check-up after treatment to ensure that you are completely cured. Don't have any sexual contacts until your doctor tells you it's safe to do so.

If you are diagnosed with gonorrhoea, it's vital that you tell all your sexual partners from the three weeks prior to your symptoms starting, and any partner since, so they may be tested and treated too.

NON-SPECIFIC URETHRITIS (NSU)

NSU is inflammation of the urethra, the tube which runs through the penis, and is the most common

STD. The germs that cause it can be present in your partner's vagina, mouth or rectum. Almost always the carrier has no symptoms and is completely unaware they are infected.

Symptoms include discomfort when urinating, which can be mild or intense, or feeling that you constantly want to pass water. There may be a cloudy discharge from the penis, which may be more noticeable in the morning.

In most cases NSU is caused by chlamydia bacteria but there are lots of other organisms that can cause it, such as thrush and herpes. Symptoms usually appear between 2–3 weeks after sexual contact with an infected person.

See your doctor as soon as you notice any symptoms. Diagnosis is made by taking a swab from the urethra. The treatment is usually a 10–14 day course of antibiotics. It's important to abstain from sexual contact and alcohol during this treatment and you should not start having sexual relations until your doctor has given you the all-clear. If this disease is left untreated, you may experience complications such as infection of the prostate or testes.

You should tell all the sexual partners you had during the incubation and infectious period so they can also be tested and treated.

CHLAMYDIA

Chlamydia is sometimes called the silent sexual disease, because people may not know they have it and if left untreated it can lead to infertility in both men and women. The chlamydia bacteria can't live outside the body, so its only means of transmission is through sexual intercourse.

In men, the symptoms may appear as inflammation of the urethra, which may cause a discharge from the penis, and/or painful or frequent urination. Inflammation of the epididymis (the thin tube leading from the testes to the vas deferens where the sperm mature) may develop, causing it to become warm, painful and swollen. This may cause infertility if untreated.

Chlamydia is difficult to detect and can only be isolated by laboratory tests. Treatment is a course of antibiotics. The full course of 10–14 days must be taken and you should have a follow-up check to ensure the disease has gone. Your sexual partners should also be treated. During treatment it is important to avoid sexual intercourse until your doctor gives you the all-clear.

GENITAL HERPES

This is a common viral infection, usually contracted through sexual contact. It's caused by the herpes simplex virus, types I and II. Either virus can infect the mouth (commonly known as cold sores) or the genital area. It is transmitted by direct, skin-to-skin contact with an infected area of another person. During oral sex the herpes virus can pass from the mouth to the genitals and vice versa.

Incubation time can vary; in the majority of cases the first outbreak will occur between 2–20 days after infection, but there are instances where symptoms take much longer to show up.

Genital herpes can affect the penis, testes, anus and the area around them. It usually appears as itchy or painful patches, or a group of tiny blisters which break, weep, then dry and usually clear up in 10–21 days. You may also feel as if you are going down with the flu, and some men also experience pain when urinating during the first occurrence.

It's important that proper diagnosis is made. This is easiest when the blisters are present and moist. There are various treatments to reduce the severity of the outbreak and frequency of attacks but, as yet, there is no cure for this disease.

You can ease the symptoms by bathing the area with salt water (1 teaspoon salt to 600ml water) twice a day, drinking plenty of water to dilute your urine, wearing loose clothing and cotton underwear and maintaining good personal hygiene. It's also important to keep the infected area dry and you can do this by using drying agents such as Betadine Cold Sore Paint, Gentian Violet and Stoxil. To relieve the pain, you can also apply Xylocaine jelly as often as necessary, to temporarily numb the area in cases of extreme discomfort and when passing urine.

If left untreated the sores will clear up by themselves, but treatment can alleviate the symptoms and help the blisters clear up faster. Abstain from sexual contact during an outbreak, as you will be at great risk of infecting your partner.

An outbreak of herpes may or may not recur. The interval between attacks may vary from more than 12 months to less than one. The virus lies dormant in the body until it is triggered, usually when your resistance is lowered by illness, sunburn, emotional stress, poor general health, tiredness or abrasion during sexual intercourse.

GENITAL WARTS

These warts are caused by the human papilloma virus and are transmitted by skin-to-skin contact during sex with an infected person. They vary in size and appearance but usually start as tiny lumps that can grow to resemble minute cauliflowers. In men they can occur on any part of the penis, scrotum and anus. They usually appear about two months after contact but may appear any time from a few weeks to 18 months later.

Genital warts are diagnosed by close examination of the skin, using magnifying equipment, after painting the area with a special solution. It's quite a painless procedure, and will show up any warts not visible to the naked eye.

Treatment is either by freezing the warts, or painting them with podophyllin paint, which needs to be applied by a doctor or nurse. Treatment is usually given 2–3 times a week for 3–4 weeks. Never buy an over-the-counter wart remover and apply it yourself, as you could do serious damage to an important part of your anatomy!

Other methods used are laser, heat treatment or surgery. Warts don't always respond to the first course of treatment, so it's important to have a check-up to ensure the problem has completely cleared up. Abstain from sex during treatment and then wear condoms to guard against re-infection. If you have genital warts, you can pass them on to your female partner. As the wart virus has been implicated in cancer of the cervix, it is particularly important that both you and your partner are diagnosed and treated.

HEPATITIS B

This disease is caused by a virus which infects the liver. Many people don't think of hepatitis B as an STD because it's usually transmitted by infected blood entering the body through injection or inoculation, such as needle sharing. But it can also be transmitted by semen, vaginal secretions, saliva or blood, entering the body through tiny scratches and abrasions. Since the virus is found in saliva, deep kissing and oral sex, as well as vaginal and anal intercourse, can result in infection.

The incubation period can be from a few weeks to several months after infection. The symptoms of hepatitis B include a general feeling of ill health, some fever, tiredness, vomiting, abdominal pains, and loss of appetite. Your skin and the whites of your eyes may turn a yellow colour (known as jaundice), but not always. Your urine may appear darker in colour and your bowel motions lighter in colour.

Early detection is important and diagnosis is made by a blood test. Once confirmed, the main form of treatment is rest, a nourishing diet and avoiding alcohol. This is a long and debilitating illness which takes many months to recover from and a small percentage of patients suffer persistent inflammation of the liver. There is a preventative vaccine which should be given to partners, but abstaining from sex is crucial during the infectious period.

If the disease is left untreated, it will usually resolve itself in about three months, but there is a risk of liver damage. You may remain infectious and become a carrier, infecting your partners unknowingly. So it's important that a correct diagnosis is made and follow-up tests taken 3–6 months later, to make sure the infection has cleared up. Blood tests should also be taken to ensure your liver has completely recovered.

All sexual partners in the six months prior to diagnosis should be tested and if you become a 'carrier' your future partners should be told, so that they can be vaccinated against the disease. Doctors and dentists should also be informed if you carry the disease and you should not donate blood.

You can reduce the risk of contracting hepatitis B by using condoms, and not sharing needles and syringes.

THRUSH

This is a fungal infection which can affect a man's foreskin and glans, causing inflammation and/or severe itching. Tight pants, stress and some antibiotics can also cause an outbreak of this infection. If you experience any discharge or itchiness in this area, consult your doctor, who can take a smear and identify the infection under a microscope.

Your doctor may prescribe a cream to apply to the affected area. You can also help control the infection by washing soon after having intercourse, and by avoiding too much soap, which can irritate the condition. You should avoid sex when your penis is inflamed.

TRICHOMONIASIS

One of the most common sexually transmitted infections, trichomoniasis is caused by germs called trichomonads. Many men carry this disease and don't realise it; others may experience a little pain in their penis and a discharge from it, or discomfort when urinating. Symptoms usually develop 1–4 weeks after sexual contact with an infected partner. If left untreated, the discharge will get steadily worse and more painful. A swab of the urethra is the quickest method of diagnosis.

Treatment consists of a single dose or a one-week course of antibiotics. You should avoid sex and alcohol until your doctor has given you the all-clear.

PUBIC LICE

Also known as 'crabs', pubic lice live in pubic hair and can be passed to other people by close physical contact, including sexual intercourse or sharing bed linen and clothing. The main symptom is an itch in your pubic hair, but it may also be in the hair of your thighs or stomach, or wherever the lice have travelled. Symptoms usually appear at least five days after contact with an infected person or bedding, but may not be noticed for up to a month.

The lice are greyish in colour and about the size of a pinhead, but their bodies may appear brownish after a meal of your blood. The adult lice are slow moving and lay their eggs on the hair shafts.

You don't have to shave off all your pubic hair to get rid of them, as was once thought. You can usually treat yourself with creams and lotions, such as Quellada or Lorexane (available over the counter at your chemist). They will kill the lice when applied directly to the pubic hair, but be careful to use these products strictly as directed on the pack. If you have a great deal of body hair, it is a good idea to apply the treatment to your whole body. After treatment, comb the hair with a very fine-toothed comb to remove the eggs from the hair shaft.

Wash all bed linen, towels and clothing in water hotter than 60°C. Repeat the process a week later to kill off any new hatchings. All current partners, plus partners from the previous four weeks and adult household members with whom close body contact or sharing of bath towels or linen may have occurred should be examined and treated.

SCABIES

Scabies is caused by mites which burrow under the skin to lay their eggs, leaving fine red marks and causing intense itching, which gets worse at night. They are passed from one person to another by direct skin contact. The mites are most commonly found in the spaces between the fingers and toes, on the wrists, and on the penis.

They can be treated easily and effectively by lotions such as Lorexane cream or Quellada lotion (available from your chemist), which should be applied according to directions, over the entire body surface from the neck down, left on overnight, then washed off thoroughly. All clothing and bed linen must be changed and washed thoroughly in water hotter than 60°C. One 24-hour application usually kills the mites, but you should repeat the process one week later.

Your partner, and all members of the household if they have it, should be treated at the same time, and all bed linen, towels and clothes should be washed.

7
What happens when you go to a sexual health centre

If you have concerns about your sexual health, you may be reluctant to go to your GP for help, because of embarrassment or because you don't wish them to become aware of your sexual activities. Perhaps you have had an extra-marital affair, or several sexual partners. Whatever the reason, you live with your fears, hoping that the problems will simply go away. Of course, they won't.

As we have seen in the chapter on sexually transmitted diseases, many symptoms will clear up without treatment, but that doesn't mean the disease has gone away, and you will still be infectious to others.

Sexual health centres have been set up in all states to cure people of STDs, quickly, confidentially and without embarrassment. What actually happens when you finally summon up the courage to walk through the door of one of these clinics?

First of all, you can phone up for an appointment without having a referral from your doctor; or you can just walk in off the street. Their services are completely free of charge and you don't need a Medicare card or health insurance to be treated. The clinics have a policy of strict confidentiality and no one other than yourself will be able to find out the results of your tests. Most people find it a great relief when they finally get to the clinic and meet the friendly, relaxed and non-judgmental staff.

THE INTERVIEW

You report to reception, fill out a registration card and are given a code. After that you will simply be called by your first name. One of the medical or nursing staff will take you to a room where a medical and sexual history will be taken and the examination will be done.

You may be feeling hostile, tense and anxious because you're insecure or embarrassed about what's happening. The staff will try to make you feel as relaxed and comfortable as they can and will make sure you know exactly what they're doing before they go ahead.

First, they need to get a general medical history, because STDs can affect the entire body in some instances. For example, syphilis and hepatitis B can have extra-genital effects, which you might not associate with a sexual health problem. It's important that you tell them all your symptoms—you may have a painful armpit or sore eyes, and not associate this with an STD.

You may find it a little embarrassing giving your sexual history but the staff have good reasons for asking the questions they do. They will need to know what your sexual practices are, so that they know what risks you've put yourself under and what STDs you might have. You'll be asked when you last had sex and when you had sex with somebody else before that. They'll also assess which of your partners will have to be contacted. For instance, if you have only been having sex with one person in the last six months, then you only need to contact one person. However, if you've had 20 contacts in the last six weeks, then you are more at risk of an STD, and your partners are also more at risk and will have to be contacted.

You may feel a little reluctant to talk about your partner/partners, but it's vitally important that you are honest—the staff will not be shocked or surprised by anything you tell them. It's not that they've heard it all before, it's just that they're open to it and comfortable with the subject. They won't look down on you or treat you as if you have done something bad. They'll just listen to what you have to say.

Some men become alarmed at the thought of having to tell their partner, but once they've seen how simple the tests and cures are for STDs, and had the consequences of not treating these diseases explained to them, most men take a responsible course of action.

The counsellor will help you work out strategies to do this, if you think it's going to be difficult. For instance, if you had a one-night stand with a girl you met in the pub and never intended to see again, the counsellor might suggest you go back to the pub on the same day of the week that you met her and she might be there again. All you'll have to do then is hand her a card, which the clinic will give you, which just says something like, 'You have been in contact with non-specific urethritis and you require treatment with an antibiotic'. She can then go to her GP, family planning clinic or sexual health centre for treatment.

THE EXAMINATION

After your history has been taken, you will be examined, have blood taken and given medication if required.

You will be asked to lie down on an examination couch, then swabs will be taken from the urethra. A urethra swab is a very fine cotton-covered stick, not unlike a cotton bud but much smaller. If the doctor is testing for gonorrhoea, the swab has to go just inside the opening of the penis to collect any secretions. If it's a chlamydia swab, it will have to be inserted two to three centimetres into the shaft of the penis, so that cells from the urethra can be collected. It sounds more horrific than it is; there is some discomfort with this test but it is not painful.

The first swab taken will be for gonorrhoea. It will be put onto a glass slide and also onto a culture plate. The results of the glass slide test will be back in 10 minutes, so you'll be told straight away if gonorrhoea has shown up and given immediate treatment. They can also tell from that slide if you have non-specific urethritis. If the slide is inconclusive, the culture plate will give a final result in three days. You'll be asked to come back and be given treatment then if necessary.

Depending on your history, other specimens will be taken and you will also be examined for genital warts and scabies. If you have a lesion, syphilis and herpes swabs will be taken—if it is caused by herpes this swab will be painful to collect because a herpes lesion is painful and that in itself is diagnostic: if it doesn't hurt then it isn't herpes. The doctor will also look for any enlarged lymph nodes in the groin, check the scrotum to see if there is any fluid retention and check that the testes are a normal size.

Also, depending on your medical and sexual history, they may test for hepatitis as well, which involves one needle prick, and from that blood sample they can test for syphilis and hepatitis B.

When you make your appointment with the clinic, you will be asked not to urinate for three hours before attending. Many men, misunderstanding this request, comply, but as soon as they enter the clinic they go to the toilet, which means the tests can't be done. If you pass urine, any discharge in your urethra is flushed away, so secretions can't be collected. So it's imperative that you do not urinate for about three hours before testing.

The clinic will *not* do a routine blood sample for HIV/AIDS. However, if your history shows risky behaviour they may recommend that you have the test, though there are certain criteria that have to be met before you can have an HIV/AIDS test. For instance, you would have to have pre-test counselling.

TREATMENT

Most STDs can be treated immediately. Gonorrhoea is treated on your first visit to the clinic. Non-specific urethritis is treated by a 10-day course of antibiotics. Syphilis, depending on the stage, is treated with a 10, 15 or 21-day course of injections. For thrush, you will be given creams to fix the problem. Hepatitis can't be treated, but your tests will show whether you are still infectious and if you are, then your partners and family should be vaccinated. You'll also be given advice on how not to spread it among your family, friends and partners.

During treatments, it's important to restrict your alcohol intake. It's also imperative that you abstain from intercourse to avoid infecting your partner. It's also advisable to stop masturbating because you have an area that has been infected and it has to rest to get better in the same way as you'd rest a sprained ankle. So give your penis a break!

Sexual health centres try to encourage people to go to them for sexual health checks before starting a new relationship. Be responsible. If you suspect that you have an STD or have been with someone who has an STD, go along to your local clinic for a check-up—it's quick, doesn't cost anything and could save you and your partner's health.

WHAT IS SAFE SEX?

The term 'safe sex' is mentioned frequently when talking about HIV/AIDS and other sexually transmitted diseases, but what we should really be talking about is 'safer sex'. Safe sex can only occur when you are in a monogamous relationship (only one partner), where neither of you has sex outside that relationship, and where neither of you is carrying the HIV/AIDS virus or an STD.

Safer sex practices will give you protection but can't provide a 100 per cent guarantee. Before starting a new relationship, it's important to check that neither of you is carrying a sexually transmitted disease, and as we mentioned before, this can be done at your local sexual health centre.

It's important to always use a condom when you have intercourse with your new partner, until you have been given the all-clear by your doctor. And if you're not sure that this new relationship is truly monogamous, or your partner hasn't had a sexual health check, continue to use condoms. If you're having sex with more than one person, then it's absolutely essential to use condoms, preferably ones that contain nonoxynol-9, as these can give added protection against HIV/AIDS and other STDs.

WHAT IS UNSAFE SEX?

Unsafe sexual practices include unprotected (not using a condom) vaginal intercourse, unprotected anal intercourse, mutual masturbation and oral sex where semen, vaginal fluid or blood comes in contact with open cuts and sores.

Remember:

- Buy good quality condoms marked with the official standards code. Check the use-by date and don't use a condom that is more than two years old.
- If you haven't used condoms before, practise on your own beforehand, to make sure you can put it on and take it off properly.
- Roll the condom onto your erect penis all the way to the base before sexual contact, being careful not to snag it on rings or with fingernails.
- Leave enough room at the tip for the semen to collect, but squeeze the tip to expel the air.
- After ejaculation, hold the rim of the condom firmly at the base of your penis as you withdraw.
- Wrap the condom in paper and throw it into the garbage bin. Do not flush it down the toilet.
- Wash and dry your penis.

Note: If you want to use a lubricant, make sure it is a water-based one like KY Jelly or Lubafax. Oil-based lubricants such as Vaseline or baby oil will make the rubber perish and therefore fail to protect you.

8
Sexual problems and solutions

Sexual problems fall into three main areas—lack of sexual desire, premature ejaculation, and impotence. The elements that create these problems are interrelated. Lack of communication with your partner, a misunderstanding of what sex is all about, and anxiety about your sexual performance are more likely causes of sexual difficulties than any medical problems.

LACK OF SEXUAL DESIRE

Loss of interest in sex can have two main causes, both of which are more mental than physical. The first is related to lifestyle, relationships and self-esteem. Today, both men and women are holding down jobs, staying on top of mortgage repayments, coping with children and trying to make a better life for themselves. It's hard for couples to share quality time where they can develop their sexual interest in one another. Sex, if it happens, tends to be a routine affair, at the end of the day after everything else has been done. There is little spontaneity and no slow seduction. With such a busy schedule, sex may seem like the final demand you just don't have the energy or the inclination to meet.

It also has a lot to do with what you *think* is expected of you and how much pressure is put on you to achieve an erection and orgasm. Let's face it, if you have worries in your life, it will affect your interest in sex.

Loss of libido could also be related to self-confidence, like failing to get an erection one time and not wanting to put yourself to the test in case it happens again. If you're worried about getting an erection you most probably won't. Once you have a goal in sex, you set up an anxiety about whether you are going to reach your goal, and the anxiety inhibits your sexual ability.

The male myths (mentioned in Chapter 1) are responsible for a lot of pressure and anxiety about sexuality. Most of the sexual information men get is based on pub gossip, locker room talk, erotic fiction and porno movies. Are you competing with some mythical man out there who's doing something— you don't even know what—that you can't do? It's amazing how many men have that nagging doubt at the back of their minds.

You may also believe that men are born with some inherent knowledge about sex, that women are not, and if you don't know about sex then you're not a man. You may feel you can't ask your friends for help, so your feelings of insecurity and inadequacy increase. Maybe you actually avoid sex altogether, so your knowledge is never tested one way or another. You may also be afraid of admitting your ignorance to your partner and so don't get help from anywhere.

Many men believe that they should get an erection at the drop of a hat (or any other item of clothing), every time the opportunity arises, no matter whether they're dead drunk, dead tired or dead worried. When they can't, they start to worry about what's wrong with them. They become increasingly concerned about getting an erection and because they're concerned, they don't. They're caught in a vicious circle.

Another pressure is the belief that women ought to have an orgasm during intercourse, and if they don't, it's the man's fault. In defence, they may taunt their partner with: 'Every other woman I've been with has managed to have an orgasm with intercourse, there must be something wrong with you!'. So, instead of just the man being anxious, the woman is too, and their sex life deteriorates even further.

The fact is that most men don't understand what stimulates women and how they reach orgasm. Those men who do seek information from sex counsellors often say they would like to know how their partner likes to be stimulated. Unfortunately, they haven't felt confident enough to ask her.

Most couples simply don't talk about what turns them on. Often women say that it is great when her partner asks her to do something for him, because it then allows her to say what she likes. Suddenly, they are able to share the experience, rather than doing it all by Braille!

Don't be conned into the belief that men should solve their own problems, and that if you ask for help you're somehow inadequate. Get it off your chest, you'll feel better for it.

The other main reason for loss of libido is due to boredom with sexual routine. You may make love in the same place, at the same time, in the same way, and it simply becomes a dreary process, so neither of you can really be bothered. If you have been with your partner for a while, you may need to experiment in doing things differently. Be more spontaneous and adventurous. It really is important for your relationship that you make some time for yourselves—just to be alone together, not necessarily to have sex but simply to talk. Again, it comes down to communicating why you don't feel like sex and being honest with one another. You'll probably find that you would both like to change the way things are, and experimenting could be a fun way to find out what you both like.

Couples with young children often worry that they are losing their sex drive. They complain that before the kids arrived they were making love all the time, but since the birth of the first one, well, they just don't feel like it any more. What these couples don't realise is that children do affect your sex life, and the time when your sex life is worst is when your children are small. Children consume an enormous amount of time and energy, and can also be emotionally draining. Is it any wonder that all you want to do is sleep when you get to bed? And when else do you get a chance to be alone? If you do start making love, sure as eggs are eggs you'll be interrupted. It's a wonder anyone ever has more than one child!

PREMATURE EJACULATION

Premature ejaculation is a term with many interpretations. Some sex therapists say it means a man who can't last in the vagina for two minutes without ejaculating; others say that it is a man who can't last long enough to satisfy his partner. Most men believe that every other man can last half an hour—but there are few women who would want them to!

As animals, we were designed to copulate quickly before a sabre-toothed tiger came along and ate us, and the human male was programmed to insert his penis, thrust a few times and then ejaculate. So the idea that the 'norm' for a man is to be able to keep thrusting away for 40 minutes is, in fact, quite unnatural.

If a couple are satisfied, it doesn't matter when ejaculation takes place. And if some men had to wait until their partner 'came', their penis would be totally worn away!

The real question is, too fast for whom? If you wish to prolong intercourse, there are techniques you can learn to achieve this. If it is your partner who wants you to last longer, in the hope that she will have an orgasm, then maybe she isn't getting the right sort of stimulation. The 'penis in vagina' is fine for climax if she is really aroused, but not much good if she's not.

The fact is that the more you worry about whether you're going to come too quickly, the more quickly you're going to come!

If you can reduce your anxiety and concern about it, then it probably won't be a problem. Consider the times when you *didn't* come too quickly. It was probably when you were relaxed and not worrying about it, or sex had occurred unexpectedly and you didn't have time to get anxious about it.

Women can sometimes add to the problem of premature ejaculation because they feel that if only the man could last longer, they would get more pleasure from intercourse, but the more the woman puts pressure on the man to last longer, the worse the problem becomes. So you really need to deal with the problem as a couple.

Sex therapists Masters and Johnson devised a 'squeeze' technique to help couples delay ejaculation. Using this method, the man's partner squeezes his penis briefly where the head joins the shaft. The slight discomfort this produces reduces the urge to ejaculate, so the couple can continue intercourse for longer.

However, many therapists today have discontinued using this method because it is a 'technique' which can add to performance anxiety. These days, they recommend a stop/start method which can be learned through masturbation. It helps the man to learn the 'point of no return', and to slow down before he gets to that point, where ejaculation is inevitable.

The next step is for the man's partner to stimulate his penis until he approaches that critical point and then stop, resuming only when the urge to ejaculate subsides. This process is repeated many times during a session and for several sessions until the man feels that he can control the timing of his ejaculation.

During intercourse, when you think you're reaching the 'point of no return', slow down or stop completely and then start again once you've regained control. You don't have to stop making love. You can continue to pleasure your partner, and stimulate her clitoris with your hand or tongue.

It's really a matter for you and your partner to work out what's going to work for you. Therapists often teach couples touching and stroking, just to increase their sensuality and to take the pressure off, and to get pleasure from genital stimulation and genital sex.

IMPOTENCE

Most men know about 'brewer's droop', when a man can't get an erection because he has had too much to drink, but did you know that obesity, smoking, marijuana, cocaine, other hard drugs and sedatives all contribute to erectile problems. If you are being treated for high blood pressure or a heart condition, the drugs may be interfering with your ability to get an erection. So consider if this could be the cause of your problem, and ask your doctor if any medication you are taking could have this side-effect.

Some men who can't get an erection still get a lot of pleasure bringing their partner to climax with their hands or mouth, but it is often the partner who is trapped with the notion that 'you're not having real sex if you don't have a penis in your vagina'.

Many women also believe they're not attractive to the man if he doesn't get a hard-on, because 'a man's erection is brought on by the sex appeal of the woman he is with'. This is simply not true. A man can find a woman immensely sexy and attractive but not get an erection for all sorts of reasons, such as concerns about work, money worries, stress, fatigue—any number of things. Ask your partner to read this book and then discuss the issue together.

If you have not been able to get or sustain an erection at some time, the best thing you can do is just forget about it. Don't set yourself the goal of having intercourse in your sex life. Realise that you can bring your partner to climax, if that's what she wants, without having to have an erection at all. You can use your hands and mouth, and for lots of women this is actually more pleasurable than intercourse. If you stop concentrating on having an erection, it will probably happen, unless there is a physical reason for it.

If you persistently fail to get an erection, or you lose it rapidly before you can have intercourse, then you should have some tests to see if there is a medical reason for this problem—it's sometimes the first sign of diabetes, or a sign of a vascular problem that should be investigated.

If it's performance anxiety, then you should just concentrate on having fun and not set yourself the goal of having intercourse. Talk to your partner about the pressure you feel to have intercourse. Explain that you'd like to have sex but basically you just want to pleasure her and have her pleasure you.

Men with impotence problems are very conscious of what their penis is doing. It's as if they are actually sitting outside themselves, watching it, and as soon as they are aware of it getting hard, they say, 'Oh, oh, is it going to stay like that? How's it doing? Oh, it's only half hard, what am I going to do?' Of course, as soon as they start thinking about it, their erection disappears.

If you find yourself doing this, start talking to your partner and get a fantasy going between you, something that will distract you; or talk about whether you are getting pleasure from what your partner is doing, rather than sitting outside your body watching to see if you are going to maintain your erection. Do anything that will take your mind off your penis and place it firmly on the sensual, stimulating feelings you are experiencing.

Unfortunately, many men with this problem hide it from their partner and instead, they avoid having sex. They also avoid all the hugging and kissing and touching that they normally would enjoy for fear that their partner will expect it to lead to intercourse and so discover their lack of erection. Consequently their partner feels rejected, often thinking she is no longer attractive to the man, or he's got another woman. This hiding of the problem creates hurt, guilt and feelings of inadequacy on both sides, which just compounds the problem. It's another vicious circle. It's devastating to the relationship because the couple may have no physical contact, communicate even less and may even feel hostile toward and suspicious of each other.

As we've said before, the tongue is a great sex aid. Try talking about your feelings. So, OK, you're not getting an erection, but that doesn't mean you can't have sex, and it's important to know that men can ejaculate and experience orgasm without an erection, if they are given the right stimulation.

Impotence may have a physical cause, but more often than not it is due to anxiety. The best way to solve the problem is, first, by talking to your partner about it, and then, if things don't improve, seeking help from the Family Planning Association. It's a common problem, but one that is usually easy to solve.

Penile implants

If you are suffering permanent impotence problems that have not responded to therapy, all is not lost. Modern medicine can do a lot these days to overcome the problem. If you can't get an erection due to a circulation disorder in your penis, there are surgical techniques which can be used to repair or bypass the damaged sections.

You could also be fitted with a penile implant. There are two main types available—one which makes the penis permanently erect, the other temporarily rigid.

To create a permanent erection, flexible plastic is inserted into the penis which allows it to bend at the appropriate angle for intercourse, but it can also be pushed to one side, to make it less obvious when not required for sex. Some men have found these a little inconvenient, because they haven't been able to hide their erection when at the beach, or dancing with their maiden aunt!

The other type of implant consists of a hydraulic arrangement that the man can inflate for intercourse, then deflate afterwards. This consists of two expandable cylinders that are implanted on both sides of the penis. These are connected to a fluid reservoir placed in the abdomen, with a pump in the scrotum. When the man wants an erection, he squeezes the pump a few times and this pumps the fluid up into the cylinders in the penis to create the erection.

You should take plenty of time to consider all the

implications before having a penile implant, because they don't come without some pain and discomfort, and as we've said before, there are other ways to have sex without intercourse.

Drug injections

Vasodilator drugs, such as Papaverine, can be injected into the penis prior to sex, which will stimulate an erection that can last for up to 40 minutes. However, this drug may have serious side-effects, so it is extremely important that you discuss all aspects of its use with your doctor. If keeping your erection is a problem, then there is also a spray containing a mild anaesthetic which can be applied to your penis before intercourse. It doesn't dull sensation but it will prolong your erection and slow down ejaculation.

If you are having impotence problems, ask your doctor to refer you to a sex therapist, or go to your local family planning clinic, which offers sex coun-selling and therapy as part of its services.

9
Sex as you grow older

Earlier in the book we dealt with the seven myths of male sexuality. Well, there is another myth that colours our attitudes towards sex and that is the myth which says: 'Sex is only for the young and beautiful'. This myth not only causes a great deal of pain and misery to young people who don't conform to the slim, smooth-muscled, beautiful image of sexual attractiveness, but also to many people past the age of 40 years.

Look at the fitness and beauty industry: these billion dollar businesses pander to our frantic attempts to stave off the ravages of time and stay as young-looking as possible, for as long as possible. Our culture dictates that sex is not for the fat, ugly, disabled, sick or old. It totally denies the fact that we are all sexual creatures and we should be able to express ourselves sexually without being made to feel ashamed or embarrassed about our needs and desires—at any age!

COMMUNITY ATTITUDES

Due to these community attitudes, older people often 'retire' from sex, in just the same way as they retire from work. They feel it's not dignified to be interested in, or have sex, at their age. 'They should have given all that up years ago.' It's particularly sad for a man or woman who loses their partner after a long and satisfying marriage where sex played a pleasurable role. They're often reluctant to seek companionship from members of the opposite sex for fear of the reaction by their family, friends and the community at large.

There's a funny aspect to human sexuality: if we feel attractive, there will be a certain 'something' about us that *is* attractive. Look what happens when we fall in love. It has a physical effect on us. Our eyes shine, our skin glows, we have a lightness to our step. It's the same with sex. If we are enjoying good sex, we are more confident, have more joy in life, are more active and interested in the world around us. This is true no matter what age we are, and older people, who are denied their natural sexuality, feel it physically too. They believe they are not sexually attractive any more, so they become less attractive. They no longer have the confidence they once had, and they may feel more frail than they actually are, because society is telling them, 'You're too old for work, you're too old for sex—you're just too old!'. It's terribly important for us as a society to change our attitudes to older people. After all, we have a vested interest in it. We are all going to be old one day!

Of course, physical changes do take place as we get older, but there is no particular age at which we should give up sex or at which sex becomes unseemly.

PHYSICAL CHANGES IN MEN

As you grow older your body produces lower levels of testosterone, your sperm count decreases, your cardiovascular and immune systems weaken and you have reduced muscle tone and general strength. At the age of 70, you wouldn't be able to beat Carl Lewis, but that doesn't mean you can't enjoy jogging. It's the same with sex!

Your testes may become smaller and more flaccid, but there is absolutely no reason why this should affect your sex life. It may take you longer to achieve an erection but, let's face it, sex is no longer a new toy and your hormones have settled down, so it's not really surprising that you don't get a hard-on all by yourself. You don't have to be responsible (at any age) for producing your erections. Let your partner have a go. She will probably enjoy taking a more active role and you can just enjoy her pleasuring you.

Your erections may not be as hard as they once were. Does it matter? Have you read Myths 1, 3 and 6 in Chapter 1? If not, go back and read them! Also, as a woman gets older, the walls of her vagina become thinner and less elastic. After menopause, she will not lubricate as much, so she may be quite content to forego the 'hard as steel' model.

As men get older the refractory period (time between erections) grows longer and it can sometimes take up to 24 hours before you become aroused again. Well, if you want sex during this period, you can have it, because as we've said over and over in this book, good sex doesn't require an erection. On the other hand, if you are having sex once every 24 hours, you'd be the envy of many much younger men!

It may take you longer to ejaculate. Human nature is perverse, isn't it? The sex clinics are full of young men worried about coming too soon and older men worried that they are not coming fast enough. The longer it takes you to ejaculate, the longer you can have intercourse, if that's what you and your partner want. Some older men won't ejaculate every time they have sex, but this means that they don't have to go through the refractory period and can have more frequent erections.

Your ejaculation will be less powerful and orgasm less intense but this doesn't seem to cause problems for most men because the sensations are just as pleasurable.

Although the sex urge comes less frequently, this doesn't have to be related to age. It can be because of sexual boredom, or the belief that 'you should have given up this nonsense years ago'. It's only very rarely that ageing causes a decline in both your interest in, and ability to have, sex. If you can go for a walk, you can enjoy sex. It is, in fact, equivalent to mild exercise and very good for you mentally, physically and emotionally.

Your children might disapprove, but so what? Look, they ruined your sex life once when they were small, so don't let them ruin it again! And anyway, it's none of their business. For some reason children can never imagine their own parents 'doing it'. Well, their children probably can't imagine them doing it either. We really do have to get away from the notion that there's a time limit on sex. If there was, you'd reach the age of sixty and, ding! your dick would drop off!

We need to fight for the right to remain real people for the whole of our lives, and that includes our right to work if we want to, have sex if we want to, have our say in society and be listened to, so that we can lead full and rewarding lives to the end.

If you have been having difficulties with sex and would like some help, talk to the Family Planning Association, who will be able to explain techniques you could use to overcome any difficulties. Read Chapters 1 and 8 again, which may also help you overcome any psychological hurdles you might have.

MEDICAL PROBLEMS

Some illnesses and medical conditions do affect your sexual ability, but to a far lesser extent than you probably imagine.

Hypertension Some men who are being treated for hypertension have reported that they have trouble gaining an erection, but this is probably due to the side-effects of the medication they are taking. If this applies to you, then consult your doctor, who may be able to change your prescription and check whether you have a vascular problem.

Diabetes About 50 per cent of men with diabetes experience difficulties with sex, even though their sexual drive is not diminished. Some suffer from impotence, others premature ejaculation. This is due to one of two causes. The first is the fact that the blood supply to the penis is gradually blocked off by cholesterol. The second is deterioration of the nerves which control the erection. If you are a diabetic, then it's important that you consult your doctor about any sexual problem you may be experiencing.

Heart disease Contrary to popular belief, there is absolutely no reason for you to avoid sex, unless advised to by your doctor. (But make sure you get a second opinion about this.) Sex is a good, mild form of exercise that can also reduce physical and emotional tension.

Prostate problems Prostate enlargement, as well as causing urinary problems, can also cause pain during erection or ejaculation. If you are experiencing these symptoms, consult your doctor for treatment.

The prostate continues to grow as you get older, but how fast it grows seems to depend on your genetic make-up. Whether the growth interferes with your urinary or sexual function also depends on which section of the gland is enlarged. In some men, a very large prostate may cause few symptoms as long as the tissue doesn't press on the urethra, but even a minor enlargement in the wrong place can cause severe problems in others. When excessive benign tissue is removed by surgery or laser treatment, potency and orgasm return to normal, but in about 50 per cent of men after surgery, the semen enters the bladder instead of the penis. This is quite harmless, but does make the man infertile.

If you have an existing medical condition and you think it may be affecting your sex life, ask your GP about it. If the doctor reassures you that it isn't a medical problem, then ask to be referred to a sex therapist or go to the Family Planning Association for advice. They're not just there to help people start a family, but to help people with all sexual matters.

10
The most commonly asked questions about sex

Q I like to masturbate at least once a day because I don't have a girlfriend at the moment. Is this normal?

A Masturbation is now recognised as a natural part of human sexuality. There is no such thing as a 'normal' number of times. You can't hurt yourself physically if you are just using your hand, and masturbation can relieve tensions in your body. There is absolutely no need for you to feel guilty. If, however, the need to masturbate many times a day is interfering with your normal life, then consult your doctor.

Q I've been told that you can lower your sperm count if you masturbate too much. Is this true? I'm 15 and I like to masturbate but I'd also like to have children when I grow up.

A Your worry stems from a schoolboy myth; it claims that men are only given so many sperm and that if they masturbate they will use them all up. This is absolute rubbish. Throughout your life your testes manufacture around 100 million sperm every day. Masturbation has no effect on your sperm production.

Q My penis doesn't hang straight, and has a slight curve to the right. Is this normal?

A Yes. It's quite common for a man's penis to hang to one side or the other. There *is* a medical condition which produces a chronic bend in the erect penis, but as you say you have a slight curve, you have nothing to worry about. However, if you are worried about it, ask your doctor to refer you to a urologist, who will be able to put your mind at ease.

Q I developed a sore on my penis, which lasted a few weeks then disappeared. I've had a few sexual partners in the last couple of months and I'm wondering if it could have been a sexually transmitted disease. I'm fine now, but I was a bit worried at the time.

A Many sexually transmitted diseases have symptoms that disappear of their own accord, while the disease remains in the body. Any sore on or near your genital area should be checked out by a doctor. If you have an STD, it is quickly and easily cured, but it's vitally important that it is diagnosed. It's also important for you to contact your sexual partners so they can be tested and treated if necessary. Don't have sexual intercourse until you have had this checked out, because you could infect others. If you are reluctant to go to your family doctor, then contact your nearest STD clinic—you'll find their number in the telephone book.

Q One of my balls hangs lower than the other. I'm worried that there may be something wrong with me.

A No, there is nothing wrong with you, it is quite normal.

Q I have a large penis, but I find most women are too small for me. I thought women were supposed to like men with big ones, but they don't seem to want to have sex with me after the first time.

A Sorry to disillusion you, but penis size is irrelevant to the enjoyment of sex. Perhaps you are not stimulating your partner enough, so that she becomes fully aroused. When a woman is aroused her vagina lengthens and becomes more elastic, ready to accept whatever size of penis is inserted. If you are entering your partner before she is ready, it's quite likely not to be a pleasant experience for her. There is a false belief among men that when a woman lubricates, she is ready for intercourse. It's not true. It only means that she is beginning to be sexually aroused, and may need far more sex play before she's really ready for intercourse. Read Chapter 1, if you haven't already.

Q I've been told that if a man doesn't have sex regularly, he gets frustrated and can become seriously ill. Is this true?

A This is often called 'blue balls' in male parlance. Sexual tensions can sometimes build up in a man who is having no sexual outlet at all, but they can easily be relieved by masturbation. However, you can't become ill from not having sex—if that was the case, no male would get past puberty! Masturbation is a natural form of sexuality and many men use this method between relationships, and even in a relationship where their partner doesn't want intercourse as often as they do.

Q Whenever my girlfriend and I have sex, I lose my erection before we can have intercourse. As soon as I feel myself becoming hard, I start to worry that it's not going to stay that way for long. Am I impotent? I don't have this problem when I masturbate.

A Worrying about losing your erection is the best way to lose it. You seem to have a performance anxiety about having to have an erection, and that if you don't, your girlfriend will think you're not a man. Just stop thinking about it. You're obviously pleasuring each other to the point of getting an erection, so as soon as your mind begins to focus on your penis, distract it by concentrating on the sexual sensations you are feeling, or get a fantasy going with your partner. It's also important to discuss this with your partner so that you don't feel that she expects you to have an erection. But the best thing is to ignore it—you'll probably find your penis won't want to be left out!

Q I think I'm losing my sex drive, because my wife wants sex much more often than I do and sometimes when we've begun to make love I just haven't been able to get it up. She says I don't love her any more, but that's not true, I do, I just don't feel like sex at the end of the day. Any suggestions?

A It's unlikely that you are losing your libido. It's probably got far more to do with what's going on in your life—work, children, money problems. If you have any worries, they will interfere with your sex life. Perhaps your days are very hassled, juggling the demands of work and home. When you get to bed, it's not surprising that you just feel like going to sleep. Perhaps your wife doesn't have as many pressures on her and so feels more receptive to sex? There could be a number of things that would put you off your stride. Remember, good sex requires relaxation, time and good communication between the partners. Make some special time just for the two of you. Get someone to look after the kids, take the phone off the hook, have a candlelight dinner, a soothing bath together, above all talk to one another and see what happens. Good sex doesn't require an erection (read Chapter 1), so just relax and have some fun.

Q I want my wife to perform oral sex on me but she refuses, saying that it's dirty. What can I do to persuade her?

A First of all, no one should make demands of their sexual partner, and they certainly shouldn't be made, or bullied, into anything they don't want to do. Have you really discussed what you both like, or would like, from sex, and why?

Ask yourself why your wife considers oral sex dirty. Are your standards of hygiene high enough? Does she realise that there are more germs in the mouth than the vagina or penis? Or does she think you might urinate or 'come' in her mouth? Does she understand how an erection works? If lack of knowledge is causing her fears, then perhaps both of you should read more about sex in general and discuss it together, or talk to a counsellor who may be able to help you both to a more rewarding sex life. However, if she is still not interested in oral sex you must respect her point of view and enjoy the other pleasures you are presently giving each other.

Glossary

Adolescence: This is the time in your life that starts with puberty and ends with adulthood.

AIDS: This term stands for Acquired Immune Deficiency Syndrome. It is a medical condition in which the body's immune system is seriously weakened. AIDS is caused by a virus called the Human Immunodeficiency Virus (HIV).

Anal sex: A form of sexual intercourse in which the penis is inserted into your partner's rectum.

Chancre: A painless sore which is one of the first symptoms of syphilis. These sores are highly contagious.

Chlamydia: A sexually transmitted disease caused by a bacteria-like organism.

Circumcision: This refers to a procedure where the foreskin is surgically removed from the head of the penis.

Clitoral hood: The tissue that extends from a woman's labia minora and forms a covering over the clitoris.

Clitoris: A small sensitive organ located in front of a woman's urethra. It is very pleasurable for most women to have their clitoris stimulated.

Coitus: A medical term for sexual intercourse.

Coitus interruptus: A means of birth control in which the penis is withdrawn from the woman's vagina before ejaculation. It is not a reliable method because sperm can be released into the vagina prior to ejaculation.

'Come': A slang term for orgasm.

Condom: A fine rubber sheath worn on an erect penis as a form of contraceptive and to prevent the spread of sexually transmitted diseases.

Contraceptive: Any device or medication that prevents pregnancy.

Cowper's glands: Two small glands connected to a man's urethra, just below the prostate gland. They produce some of the fluid that emanates from the penis prior to ejaculation.

Cunnilingus: Oral sex play where the man stimulates the woman's vulva with his tongue.

Ejaculation: When semen spurts from the man's penis at the time of orgasm.

Epididymis: A thin tube leading from the testes to the vas deferens.

Erection: When the penis becomes engorged with blood, making the penis stiff and erect.

Erogenous zones: Areas of the body that are sensitive

to sexual excitement, such as the lips, breasts and genitals.

Erotic: Anything that causes sexual arousal, such as fiction, movies, clothing, etc.

Fellatio: A type of oral sex where the woman stimulates the man's penis with her mouth.

Female superior position: This is a position in intercourse where the woman lies on top of and facing the man.

Fertility: Your ability to produce children.

Foreplay: Any sexual play.

Foreskin: The skin that covers the head of the penis in uncircumcised males.

Genital herpes: A sexually transmitted disease. It is caused by a viral infection and symptoms include painful blisters and sores around the genital area.

Genitals: The external sexual organs.

Glans: The head of the penis.

Gonorrhoea: A sexually transmitted disease caused by a bacterial infection. It is easily treated with antibiotics, but can be serious if left untreated.

Gynaecomastia: A temporary enlargement of a boy's breasts during puberty.

'Hard-on': A slang term for an erection.

Hepatitis: A debilitating infection of the liver, often transmitted sexually.

Impotence: When a man is unable to gain an erection.

Infertility: The inability to have children.

'Jerking off': A slang term for masturbation.

Labia: The lips of a woman's genitals. There are two

sets, the labia majora (the outer lips) and the labia minora (the inner lips).

Lateral position: A position in sexual intercourse in which the couple lie side by side, facing each other.

Male superior position: Commonly known as the missionary position, this is when the man lies on top of the woman, facing her.

Masturbation: Touching your genital organs to produce sexual excitement and orgasm.

Nocturnal emissions: Also known as 'wet dreams', this is when a boy ejaculates involuntarily in his sleep. It is a very common occurrence in pubescent boys. There is nothing you can do to prevent it and it is perfectly natural.

Oral sex: This is when a man or a woman stimulates his or her partner's genitals with their mouth.

Orgasm: The peak of sexual excitement that results in a climax, and ejaculation in men.

Penis: The male organ for urination and sexual activities.

Premature ejaculation: When a man can't control the timing of his ejaculation. It should not be confused with the 'point of no return' when ejaculation becomes inevitable.

Prostate gland: A gland in men that surrounds the urethra, where the vas deferens join the urethra, just below the bladder. It produces the seminal fluid.

Penile prothesis: A permanent implant in a man's penis that enables him to have an erection.

Puberty: The time when a boy matures physically and sexually.

Pubic area: The area of the body which surrounds the genital organs.

Pubic hair: The hair that grows in the pubic area.

Pubic lice (crabs): Small parasites that live in pubic hair and which can be spread sexually.

Refractory period: The period after ejaculation during which a man is incapable of gaining another erection.

Scrotum: The sac of skin that contains the testes.

Semen: The thick, whitish fluid that spurts from the penis during ejaculation.

Seminal fluid: The fluid in which the sperm are suspended.

Seminal vesicles: These are small sac-like structures at the end of each vas deferens. They are situated near the bladder, and produce most of the seminal fluid.

Sexual intercourse: When a man places his penis into the woman's vagina during sex.

Sexually transmitted disease (STD): Any disease that is spread through sexual activity.

Shaft: The longer part of the penis.

Sixty-nine (69): A position where a couple mutually stimulate one another's genitals with their mouths.

Sperm: The male reproductive cells.

Spermicide: A cream, lotion or jelly that is inserted into the vagina to kill sperm.

Syphilis: A highly contagious sexually transmitted disease. If left untreated, it can cause serious, long-lasting damage to your health, or even death.

Testes: Also called testicles, these are the two small

oval male sex glands located in the scrotum. They produce the sperm and male sex hormones.

Testosterone: The main male sex hormone.

Trichomonasis: A sexually transmitted disease that may have no symptoms in the male even though he is carrying it.

Urethra: The tube which passes through the penis, through which you urinate and ejaculate.

Vagina: The passage leading from the uterus to the vulva in the female.

Vulva: The external female genitals, specifically the two pairs of labia and the cleft between them.

Vasa deferentia (sing. vas deferens): Two tubes which carry the sperm from the epididymis, through the prostate gland to enter the urethra.

Vasectomy: Male sterilisation operation where the vas deferens are cut and tied off so that sperm cannot mix with the semen.

Wet dreams: See Nocturnal emissions.

Withdrawal: See Coitus interruptus.